SLEEP BLİSS

Unlocking Sweet Dreams in the Modern Parenting Journey

By

Edwina M. Byrd

Table contents

Copyright

© [2023] [Edwina M. Byrd]

İntroduction

Enter the world of "Sleep Bliss:Unlocking Sweet Dreams in the Modern Parenting Journey where the scent of possibilities lingers. Consider an exhausted but optimistic new mom traversing the maze of restless nights, longing for a break. That mother was me. I discovered this transforming guide among the nighttime whispers and nursery shadows.

The first few pages were a surprise, promising that sleep did not have to be a distant memory. A symphony of transformation unfurled as I submerged myself in its teachings. My baby's screams subsided into a peaceful sleep as bedtime became a lovely journey. The effect lasted beyond our evenings, filling each day with renewed vigor and excitement.

I developed a strategy for recovering my rest and appreciating the wonder of parenthood. This is more than a book; it's a lifeline to more peaceful evenings and brighter mornings. If you're looking for a change, this book is your passport to a trip where sleep is no longer a luxury but a lovely reality just waiting to be discovered.

CHAPTER 1

CHİLD REST BASİCS

Establishing a Quiet Rest Climate

Investigate the meaning of a helpful rest climate for your child, covering variables like encompassing lighting, open-to-bedding, and room temperature. Figure out how to work out some kind of harmony to make a quiet haven for peaceful evenings. A quiet rest climate is urgent for your child's prosperity, making way for helpful and continuous rest. Investigate the accompanying angles to guarantee you've made the ideal rest safe haven:

- Surrounding Lighting: Delicate, faint lighting during sleep time helps signal to your child that now is the ideal time to slow down. Consider utilizing a nightlight with a warm sparkle to make a mitigating air.
- Open to Bedding: Pick comfortable and breathable sheet material to control your child's temperature. Choose delicate, hypoallergenic textures that give an agreeable rest surface.
- Room Temperature: Keep a moderate room temperature, commonly between 68-72°F (20-22°C). Dress your child in layers to adapt to temperature vacillations and guarantee they're neither too hot nor excessively cold.

- Repetitive sound Children's songs: Delicate, reliable foundation sounds can cover family commotions and create a quiet feeling. Investigate choices like repetitive sounds or delicate bedtime songs to calm your child into a tranquil sleep.
- Clean up and Streamline: Keep the rest space straightforward and liberated from interruptions. A messiness-free climate limits feeling and advances a feeling of smoothness.
- Comfortable Rest Space: Assign an agreeable and safe rest region for your child. A den with a solid sleeping cushion and fitted sheet is great. Abstain from delicate sheet material, toys, or free things that could represent a danger.
- Customized Contacts: Consider adding individual contacts, like an encouraging cover or a recognizable toy. These things can give a feeling of safety to your child.

Keep in mind, that the objective is to establish a climate that elevates unwinding and indicates to your child that it's the ideal opportunity for rest. By focusing on these subtleties, you're encouraging sound rest propensities as well as sustaining a feeling of safety and solace that will add to a good rest insight for your little one.

Laying out a Predictable Sleep Schedule

Jump into the significance of consistency in sleep time schedules. Laying out a reliable sleep time routine is a foundation for advancing solid rest for your child. Make a quieting succession of exercises, like a steaming shower, delicate cradlesongs, or a tranquil story. Reiteration of these ceremonies signs to your child that now is the right time to slow down, cultivating a feeling of safety and consistency. Keep the normal basic, calming, and reliable to help your little one change flawlessly from attentiveness to rest, making way for serene evenings of rest.

Enveloped by Solace

Dig into the specialty of wrapping up, a revered strategy that impersonates the cozy impression of the belly. Find the advantages, legitimate wrapping-up strategies, and when to change away from wrap-up as your child develops.

The specialty of wrapping up is a revered method that includes cozily enclosing your child with a cover, establishing a protected and case-like climate. This training impersonates the impression of being in the belly, giving solace and advancing better rest. When done accurately, wrapping up can assist with forestalling the surprise reflex, permitting your child to rest all the more adequately. It's crucial to utilize lightweight, breathable textures and guarantee that the wrap-up is cozy yet not excessively close, taking into account legitimate hip development. As your child develops, be mindful of indications of status to progress away from wrapping up for protected and agreeable rest.

Understanding Rest Prompts and Examples

Understanding your child's rest prompts and examples is a vital part of responsive nurturing. Investigate the unpretentious prompts and examples your child displays, assisting you with understanding their extraordinary rest needs. From tired signs to perceiving different rest cycles, gain bits of knowledge into the language of your child's rest.

> ➢ Sleepy Signs: Perceive unobtrusive indications of sluggishness, like diminished action, more slow developments, and saggy eyelids. Getting these signs early is considered a smoother progress into rest.

> ➢ Taking care of Signs: Comprehend how your child's taking care of examples is interlaced with rest. Perceive hunger prompts and lay out a care schedule that supplements rest cycles, advancing better rest.

> ➢ Rest Wake Cycles: Infants experience more limited rest cycles than grown-ups. Find out about the normal term of these cycles and how to

answer enlightenments to energize self-alleviating and longer times of rest.

> ➤ Day-Night Separation: Assist your child with laying out a circadian mood by presenting them to normal light during the day and making a faint, calm climate around evening time. This guides them in controlling their rest wake cycle.

> ➤ Adaptability: Infants' rest needs to advance as they develop. Remain mindful of changes in rest designs during formative achievements, getting teeth, or ailment, and change schedules in like manner.

> ➤ Make a Rest Log: Keep a straightforward rest log to follow your child's rest prompts, examples, and evening time enlightenments. This can give important bits of knowledge about their extraordinary rest needs and assist you with fitting schedules.

Understanding these signs and examples engages you to answer speedily and punctually to your child's rest needs. By tuning into their signs, you can establish a strong rest climate that supports sound rest propensities from the earliest phases of life.

Exploring Rest Relapses and Achievements

Expect and beat normal rest relapses as your child arrives at different formative achievements. Outfit yourself with techniques to explore these transitory disturbances and back your child's advancing rest needs.

- ❖ Perceiving Rest Relapses: Comprehend that rest relapses are brief disturbances in rest designs frequently connected with formative jumps. Normal relapse periods incorporate about 4 months, 8-10 months, and a year and a half. Anticipate brief changes in rest conduct during these times.

- ❖ Solace and Consistency: During relapses, give additional solace and keep up with consistency in sleep time schedules. Console your child with natural rest signs to assist them with exploring through the transitory disturbance.

- ❖ Development Sprays: Perceive that development sprays can concur with rest relapses. During these times, your child might encounter expanded hunger, prompting more successive evening feedings. Be receptive to their healthful requirements.

- ❖ Getting teeth Difficulties: Getting teeth can disturb rest because of distress. Integrate calming teeth cures into your everyday practice, for example, chilled getting teeth toys or delicate back rubs, to reduce distress and advance better rest.

- ❖ Observing Achievements: Recognize and celebrate formative achievements, for example, turning over, sitting up, or creeping. These accomplishments can briefly influence rest as your child rehearses new abilities. Offer consolation during alert times and change rest schedules on a case-by-case basis.
- ❖ Tolerance and Adaptability: Embrace tolerance and adaptability during these stages. Comprehend that relapses are a characteristic piece of improvement, and with your help, your child will adjust to new abilities and dozing designs.

By perceiving the rhythmic movement of rest relapses and achievements, you can move toward these stages with a proactive and versatile mentality. Your responsiveness and understanding assume an urgent part in assisting your child to explore these changes with no sweat as could really be expected.

Rest Security Rules

Making a Safe Rest Space: Focus on your child's well-being during rest by getting it and executing fundamental security rules. From safe rest positions to lodging wellbeing, guarantee that your child dozes sufficiently in a protected climate. Continuously put your child on their back to rest, as this position diminishes the gamble of Sudden Infant Death Syndrome (SIDS). This suggestion applies to the two rests and evening rest. Furnish a solid sleeping cushion with a fitted sheet in the house. Abstain from delicate sheet material, guard cushions, or toys, as they present suffocation chances. The rest space ought to be moderate and liberated from expected perils. Consider room sharing without bed sharing. Place your bassinet or bassinet close to your bed for the initial half year to a year. This closeness takes into consideration simple observing and encouraging. Dress your child in lightweight, breathable layers to forestall overheating. Keep the room temperature moderate, and try not to utilize weighty covers or blankets. Present a pacifier at naptime and sleep time. Research recommends that pacifier use might lessen the gamble of SIDS. In any case, if breastfeeding, hold on until breastfeeding is deep-rooted before presenting a pacifier. Keep the rest climate without smoke. Openness to tobacco smoke, in any event, during pregnancy, builds the gamble of SIDS. Abstain from smoking or vaping close to your child's rest space. Go to ordinary well-child exams to screen your child's development and improvement. Examine any worries about rest and well-being with your medical care supplier. Assuming that you decide to wrap up, guarantee it's done securely. Utilize lightweight, breathable covers, and pass on sufficient space for your child's hips to move. Cease wrapping up once your child gives indications of turning over.

Complying with these rest well-being rules gives a protected rest climate to your child, advancing their prosperity and diminishing the gamble of rest-related mishaps. Continuously talk with your medical services supplier for customized direction in light of your child's one-of-a-kind requirements and conditions.

Investigating Normal Rest Difficulties

Tending to normal rest difficulties requires a smart and versatile methodology.

- Rest Hardships: Issues with snoozing can frequently be connected to overtiredness or under-sluggishness. Lay out a steady rest plan, make a quieting pre-rest schedule, and guarantee a climate helpful for rest.
- Changing to a Bunk: In the event that your child is progressing from a bassinet to a den, make the new rest space recognizable by setting natural items, and step by step expand the time spent in the bunk during conscious periods to fabricate positive affiliations.
- Getting teeth Uneasiness: Getting teeth can upset rest. Give calming cures, for example, getting teeth toys, chilled washcloths, or delicate back rubs before sleep time. Think about offering

relief from discomfort as exhorted by your medical care supplier.

- Laying out a Sleep time Schedule: On the off chance that your child battles with sleep time, return to and change your sleep time schedule. Guarantee consistency, consolidate quieting exercises, and make an anticipated succession to flag that rest is drawing nearer.

- Establishing an Agreeable Rest Climate: Assess the rest climate for expected inconvenience. Check for legitimate room temperature, change clothing layers as needed, and guarantee the den sleeping pad is agreeable and strong.

- Answering Bad Dreams or Night Dread: Separate between bad dreams and night fear. Bad dreams might require ameliorating, while night fear generally resolves all alone. Give consolation without completely waking your child during night fear.

Keep in mind, that investigating rest difficulties is a continuous cycle that requires persistence and perception. Tailor your methodology in view of your child's exceptional disposition and needs, and talk with medical services experts assuming that difficulties endure or arise.

CHAPTER 2

TYPİCAL INFANT REST SCHEDULE

Rest Term and Examples

Comprehend the ordinary rest examples of an infant, including incessant waking, short rest cycles, and an absence of an unmistakable day-night cadence. Perceive that infants rest for more limited spans, going from 14 to 17 hours per day.

Taking care of and Rest Affiliation

Investigate the association among taking care of and rest for infants. Perceive the job of yearning in evening time arousals and comprehend how babies frequently partner taking care of with nodding off.

Day-Night Disarray

Recognize the peculiarity of day-night disarray in babies. Learn systems to assist with laying out a day-night musicality, for example, presenting your child to regular light during the day and keeping evening cooperations quiet and calm.

Rest Climate

Establish a protected and helpful rest climate for your infant. Stress the significance of putting your child on their back to rest, guaranteeing a solid sleeping pad, and abstaining from delicate sheet material, toys, or free things in the bunk.

Wrapping up Strategies

Investigate the advantages of wrapping up as a relieving procedure for infants. Gain proficiency with the appropriate wrapping-up methods utilizing lightweight, breathable covers, and comprehend when to change away from wrapping up as your child develops.

Infant Rest Signs

Perceive the unpretentious signs that show your infant is prepared for rest. From yawning and scouring eyes to getting some distance from feeling, understanding these signs can assist you with starting the sleep time routine brilliantly.

Rest Relapse and Development Sprays

Expect rest relapses and development sprays in the early months. Perceive that impermanent disturbances in rest are normal during formative jumps and development sprays, and learn techniques to explore these periods.

Making a Sleep Time Schedule

Lay out a delicate sleep time routine to indicate to your infant that now is the right time to rest. Investigate quieting exercises like a steaming shower, delicate cradlesongs, or perusing a delicate story as business as usual.

Solace and Alleviating Strategies

Find successful alleviating strategies for your infant. From delicate shaking and influencing to utilizing repetitive sound as a pacifier, comprehend how to establish a consoling climate that energizes serene rest.

Understanding what is ordinary in infant rest includes perceiving the fluctuation in rest designs, executing safe rest rehearses, and being receptive to your child's singular necessities. By embracing these perspectives, you can encourage a positive rest climate for your infant.

CHAPTER 3

NORMAL SLEEP TİME SLİP-UPS AND ARRANGEMENT

1. Sleep time Opposition: Your youngster opposes heading to sleep, prompting sleep time fights. Lay out a steady sleep schedule, establish a quiet climate, and address any feelings of dread or tension. Include your youngster in picking components of the daily schedule to encourage a feeling of control.

2. Night Wakings: assuming your youngster wakes oftentimes during the evening, upsetting their rest. Assess and address potential causes like inconvenience, hunger, or conflicting sleep time schedules. Empower self-alleviating by permitting brief periods prior to meditating, progressively stretching out as your youngster turns out to be more autonomous.

3. Trouble Nodding off Alone: Your kid battles to nod off without your presence. Slowly change from remaining with your kid until they nod off to empowering self-relieving. Present solace things or a unique sleep time toy to give consolation.

4. Apprehension about Dull or Bad Dreams: Feeling of dread toward dim or bad dreams causes sleep

time tension. Use nightlights, offer a solace object, and approve your kid's sentiments. Make a sleep schedule that incorporates quieting exercises and addresses particular feelings of trepidation through open correspondence.

5. Conflicting Sleep time: Sleep time changes, prompting disarray and rest interruptions. Lay out a reliable sleep time and routine to flag when now is the right time to slow down. Consistency directs your kid's interior clock and advances a smoother sleep time insight.

6. Innovation Impedance: Screen time before bed influences rest quality. Carry out a without-screen wind-down period before sleep time. Energize loosening up exercises like perusing or paying attention to quieting music as opposed to drawing in with electronic gadgets.

7. Overtiredness: Your youngster becomes overtired, making it harder for them to settle down. Guarantee an age-fitting sleep time that considers sufficient rest. Focus on your kid's rest prompts and change sleep time on a case-by-case basis to forestall overtiredness. Stretched-out attentiveness can prompt trouble nodding off. Guarantee age-proper sleep times, and keep a predictable rest plan.

8. Progressing to a Major Youngster Bed: Moving from a den to a bed presents difficulties. Steadily

present the possibility of a major youngster bed. Permit your youngster to be important for the interaction by picking bedding or another bed. Build up a certain relationship with the new rest space.

9. Rest Affiliations: Your youngster depends on unambiguous circumstances to nod off. Empower free rest by slowly decreasing rest affiliations. The shift from being available until your youngster nods off to permitting them to self-relieve. Consistency is vital.

Tending to these normal sleep time issues includes persistence, consistency, and grasping your kid's singular necessities. Tailor answers to fit your youngster's demeanor and inclinations, making a sleep schedule that cultivates a positive and tranquil rest insight.

CHAPTER 4

UNDERSTANDİNG EVENİNG TİME TAKİNG CARE OF İN CHİLDREN

★ Dietary Necessities

Perceive that evening time feedings serve an urgent job in gathering your child's dietary requirements, particularly during the early months. Infants have little stomach limits, and successive feedings assist with giving the essential calories for development and advancement.

★ Solace and Security

Recognize the job of evening-time nursing as a wellspring of solace and security for your child. Past sustenance, the nearby actual contact, and the relieving nature of breastfeeding add to a feeling of profound prosperity and connection.

★ Development Sprays

Comprehend that children frequently experience development sprays, during which they might display expanded cravings and more incessant evening arousals. These stages are impermanent, and answering your child's expanded craving upholds a solid turn of events.

★ Formative Changes

Know about formative changes that might impact evening time taking care of examples. Getting teeth, formative jumps, and expanded versatility can influence rest, prompting more successive night feedings as your child explores these achievements.

★ Breast Milk Arrangement

Comprehend that the synthesis of bosom milk changes constantly. Evening bosom milk contains more significant levels of specific parts, for example, melatonin, which might add to a quieting impact and help in advancing rest.

★ Parental Solace and Holding

Perceive that evening time feedings are a chance for parental solace and holding. These calm, cozy minutes encourage areas of strength among you and your child, adding to a feeling that everything is good and trust.

★ Continuous Changes in Rest Patterns

The value that as your child develops, rest designs normally advance. Progressive changes in evening time taking care of and dozing designs are essential for the formative cycle. Urge a responsive way to deal with your child's evolving needs.

★ Social and Individual Varieties

Comprehend that evening time taking care of practices can change across societies and among individual families. Social standards, relational peculiarities, and individual inclinations assume a part in molding evening time to take care of schedules.

★ Adjusting Rest Needs

Make progress toward harmony between meeting your child's wholesome and profound requirements during evening time feedings while likewise considering the significance of advancing sound rest propensities. Progressive changes and responsive nurturing can assist with finding some kind of harmony.

Exploring evening taking care requires a comprehension of both the viable and close-to-home viewpoints included. Embrace the uniqueness of your child's requirements, look for help when required, and move toward evening feedings as an all-encompassing part of your providing care venture.

Why Infants Eat Around Evening Time

Babies and newborn children frequently awaken around evening time to take care of because of their small stomach limit and fast development. Evening feedings give fundamental supplements and add to sound weight gain. Furthermore, infants might utilize evening time nursing as a wellspring of solace and consolation, looking for the nearby association with their parental figure during these weak hours.

At the point when the Child is Ravenous

Perceiving hunger signals is significant for responsive nurturing. Indications of appetite incorporate establishing, sucking on clenched hands, expanded sharpness, and general fretfulness. It's vital to answer expeditiously to these prompts, guaranteeing your child gets the sustenance they need.

Late evening Dietary pattern

A few children foster an evening-time dietary pattern that goes past wholesome necessities. This propensity can be connected to comfort, mitigating, or dependence on nursing to fall back on snoozing. While this conduct is normal, it can present difficulties for the two guardians and the child when it turns into a delayed example.

Late Evening Weaning Procedures

Late evening weaning includes slowly diminishing or taking out evening feedings to energize longer stretches of rest. Begin by guaranteeing your child is very much taken care of during the day to address dietary issues. Acquaint a reliable sleep time routine by laying out clear rest affiliations. Progressively decline the term of evening time takes care of or acquaint mitigating strategies with the assistance your child figure out how to self-relieve.

Normal Issues in Evening Weaning

- Protection from Change: Infants might oppose changes to their evening schedule. Be patient and present changes bit by bit.
- Getting teeth or Inconvenience: Getting teeth or distress can upset rest and lead to expanded evening feedings. Address these issues with fitting cures.
- Irregularity in Approach: Consistency is key in evening weaning. Irregularity in your methodology might befuddle your child. Adhere to an arrangement and show restraint toward the cycle.
- Close-to-home Solace: Babies frequently partner evening nursing with close-to-home solace. Present option alleviating procedures and guarantee your child has a good sense of reassurance in alternate ways.
- Parental Agreement: Guarantee that guardians or parental figures are in total agreement concerning late evening weaning techniques. Reliable methodologies from all parental figures add to a smoother change.

Exploring the harmony between evening time taking care of and rest is an individual excursion, and each child is remarkable. Focus on your child's signals, embrace a responsive methodology, and consider talking with a medical care proficient for direction custom-fitted to your child's singular requirements.

CHAPTER 5

NORMAL REST DİFFİCULTİES

1) Rest Relapse: Unexpected disturbances in rest designs, frequently happening around formative achievements or changes. Comprehend that rest relapses are transitory. Keep up with consistency in schedules, give solace, and be patient as your child acclimates to new formative stages.

2) Progressing to a Major Youngster Bed: Moving from a lodging to a bed might upset rest schedules. Bit by bit present the new bed, include your youngster in the change cycle, and keep a reliable sleep time routine to facilitate the change.

3) Fear of abandonment: Dread or misery when isolated from parental figures, particularly at sleep time. Foster a consoling sleep schedule, use solace things, and proposition delicate consolation. Step by step broaden the time spent away, supporting the message that you'll return.

4) Overstimulation Before Bed: Inordinate feelings before sleep time can prompt trouble settling down. Establish a tranquil and faint climate paving the way to sleep time. Limit screen time

and invigorating exercises to assist your kid with changing to a more loosened-up state.

5) Sickness or Uneasiness: Infection, distress, or torment can disrupt rest. Give additional solace, change rest positions if necessary, and guarantee fitting clinical consideration. Establish a calming climate to advance rest during sickness.

Exploring normal rest misfortunes includes a mix of figuring out your youngster's novel requirements, keeping up with consistency in schedules, and answering with persistence and consolation. Addressing these difficulties with an insightful methodology adds to the foundation of sound rest propensities for your youngster.

Guaranteeing the prosperity of a child's rest is fundamental, and there are potential unexpected problems that guardians ought to know about. While these confusions are not comprehensive, they feature critical worries that might influence a child's rest and general well-being.

Likely unexpected problems with snoozing infants

Rest Apnea

Rest apnea in children includes brief breaks in breathing during rest. It tends to be brought about by variables like broadened tonsils or adenoids. Rest apnea can prompt insufficient oxygen levels, influencing development and improvement. It might bring about daytime drowsiness, peevishness, and potential long-term medical problems whenever left untreated.

Reflux or GERD (Gastroesophageal Reflux Sickness)

GERD happens when the stomach corrosive streams once more into the throat, causing distress. This can be especially articulated during resting. Children with GERD might encounter disturbed rest because of inconvenience or agony, prompting continuous evening time arousals. Tending to GERD through clinical direction is vital for further developing the best quality.

Related Breathing Issues

Conditions like bronchopulmonary dysplasia or innate heart deformities can affect breathing during rest. These issues might prompt sporadic breathing examples, stops in breathing, or expanded work of relaxing. Legitimate clinical administration is fundamental for addressing the basic circumstances and backing solid rest.

Rest Development Issues

Messes like fretful leg condition or intermittent appendage development turmoil can cause compulsory developments during rest. These developments might upset rest and lead to daytime drowsiness. Recognizing and overseeing development problems can add to further developed rest quality.

Rest Related Seizures

A few children might encounter seizures during rest, known as nighttime seizures. Seizures can cause disturbances in rest, affecting generally rest engineering. Distinguishing and dealing with the basic reasons for nighttime seizures is essential for a child's prosperity.

Rest Related Development Issues (SRMD)

Conditions like childish fits or late evening waking issues fall under this class. SRMD can prompt disturbances in rest, influencing both the span and nature of rest. Convenient clinical mediation is important to address these problems.

Rest Problems Related to Neurological Circumstances

Neurological circumstances, for example, cerebral paralysis or formative deferral can affect rest. These circumstances might add to difficulties in nodding off, staying unconscious, or keeping a steady rest plan. Tending to the neurological viewpoints is indispensable for supporting sound rest designs.

Contaminations and Respiratory Issues

Respiratory contaminations, for example, respiratory syncytial infection (RSV) or pneumonia, can influence breathing during rest. Respiratory issues might prompt upset rest, expanded arousal, and likely complexities on the off chance that respiratory pain happens. Clinical consideration is critical for dealing with these circumstances.

Guardians ought to be cautious and talk with medical services experts assuming that they notice persevering rest aggravations or any unsettling ways of behaving in their child's rest. Early location and mediation assume a key part in tending to likely unexpected problems and advancing ideal rest and generally speaking well-being.

Conclusion

We wind up on an excursion enlightened by recently discovered information and bits of knowledge into the sensitive domain of newborn child rest. From understanding the complexities of evening time taking care to explore normal difficulties, we've dove into the workmanship and study of encouraging quiet evenings for the two infants and guardians. As we close this part, how about we ponder the force of responsive nurturing, the meaning of laying out schedules, and the steadfast love that supports each rest-related challenge? " Rest Happiness" isn't simply an aide; it's an ally for the sleepless evenings, a guide for the questionable minutes, and a demonstration of the strength of being a parent. May these common encounters and master experiences make ready for peaceful evenings, making an embroidery of loved recollections and encouraging the rest happiness each family merits. Here's to relaxing evenings, flourishing families, and the persevering through excursion of being a parent. Rest soundly, think beyond practical boundaries, and embrace the delighted minutes that each new first light brings.

www.ingramcontent.com/pod-product-compliance
Lightning Source LLC
Chambersburg PA
CBHW070753260726
48660CB00007B/3093